The Benefits of Pomegranate
Fruit From Jannah Paradise
For Mental Health & Body Healing

by

Jannah Firdaus Mediapro

2021

The Benefits of Pomegranate Fruit from Jannah Paradise For Mental Health & Body Healing

JANNAH FIRDAUS MEDIAPRO

PUBLISHING

2021

The Benefits of Pomegranate Fruit from Jannah Paradise
For Mental Health & Body Healing

Prologue

The pomegranate is a fruit-bearing deciduous shrub in the family Lythraceae, subfamily Punicoideae that grows between 5 and 10 m tall. The pomegranate was originally described throughout the Mediterranean region.

The fruit is typically in season in the Northern Hemisphere from October to Februaryand in the Southern Hemisphere from March to May. As intact sarcotestas or juice, pomegranates are used in baking, cooking, juice blends, meal garnishes, and smoothies.

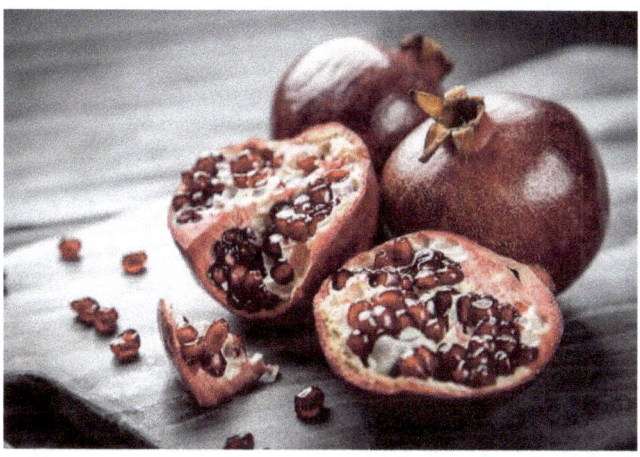

Pomegranates are widely cultivated throughout the Middle East and Caucasus region, north and tropical Africa, the Indian subcontinent, Central Asia, the drier parts of Southeast Asia, and the Mediterranean Basin.

The Benefits of Pomegranate Fruit from Jannah Paradise
For Mental Health & Body Healing

Fresh juice doesn't have to be green or full of spinach to be healthy. Pomegranate juice contains more than 100 phytochemicals. The pomegranate fruit has been used for thousands of years as medicine.

Today, pomegranate juice is being studied for its many health benefits. It may help with cancer prevention, immune support, energy boost, antivirus and fertility.

Pomegranate Fruit from Jannah Paradise

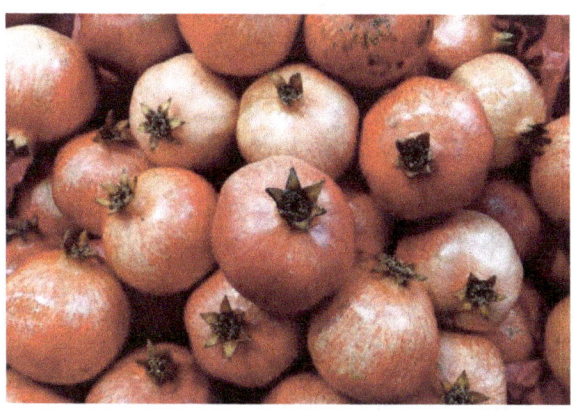

Allah SWT (God) Say:

"He is the One who sent down water from the heavens. Then We brought forth with it vegetation of all kinds. Then from it We brought grains set upon one another.

From the palm-trees, from their spathes, come forth the low hanging bunches. (We produce) vineyards and the olive and the pomegranate, either similar or not similar to each other.

Look at its fruit when it bears fruit, and at its ripening. Surely, in all this there are signs for the people who believe"

(The Noble Quran Surah 6 Verse 99)

Prophet Muhammad SAW told his companions that each pomegranate potentially held a heavenly grain, "There is not a pomegranate which does not have a pip from one of the pomegranate of the Garden (Jannah) in it."

(Sahih Hadith Bukhari & Muslim)

Pomegranates are one of the paradise fruits mentioned in The Holy Quran.

Quranic medicine scholars believe that pomegranate as a fruit of paradise comes in autumn.

Because the autumn season is the fall season of trees and clogs of the sky and is very useful in preventing depression and worry.

Pomegranate Fruit Can Reassure The Heart & Soul

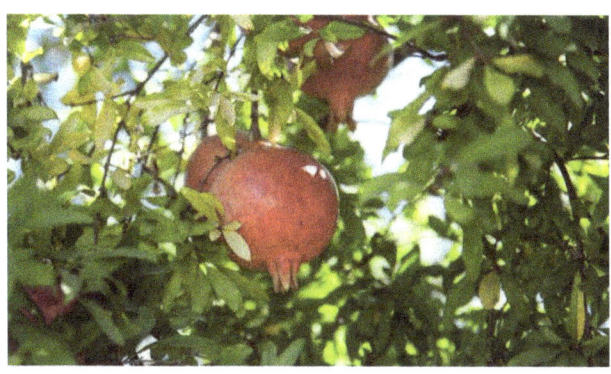

Prophet Muhammad (PBUH) said: Eat pomegranate because its grain cleanse your heart and removes the devil from the body for 40 days.

Prophet Muhammad (PBUH) said: Whoever eats pomegranate, his heart becomes clear and temptation leaves him for 40 days.

Prophet Muhammad (PBUH) said: Whoever eats a whole pomegranate God enlightens his heart for 40 days.

Prophet Muhammad (PBUH) said: Eat pomegranate with its peel because it cleanses your stomach.

Prophet Muhammad (PBUH) said: Pomegranate is above all fruits and whoever eats a pomegranate makes his devil angry for 40 nights.

Amir al-Mu'minin Imam Ali ibn Abu Talib (AZ) said: There is a of heart and self- light in every pomegranate seed that falls in the stomach and makes the devil of obsession sick for 40 nights.

Pomegranate Fruit For Stress Relief & Improve Mental Health Healing

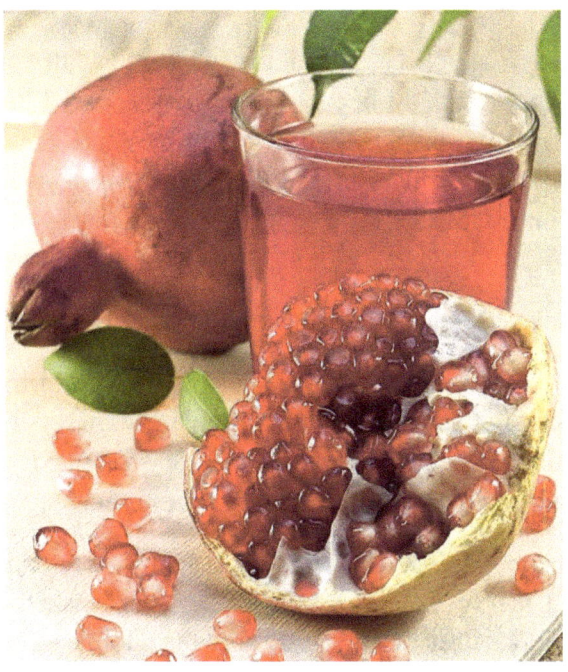

Fresh juice doesn't have to be green or full of spinach to be healthy. Pomegranate juice contains more than 100 phytochemicals. The pomegranate fruit has been used for thousands of years as medicine.

Having a daily consumption of pomegranate juice could help to eliminate stress in the office as well as helping people to love their job.

A new study has found pomegranate juice causes a significant reduction in levels of the stress hormone cortisol and also lowers blood pressure.

Recent research has found that 41 percent of workers in Britain claim to be stressed or very stressed in their jobs and two-thirds of workers said they feel they have been put under more pressure by management since the economic downturn.

However, pomegranate juice can help to make employees feel more enthusiastic about their work.

Sixty volunteers took part in the study which was carried out by the Queen Margaret University in Edinburgh, Scotland, to assess the physiological effect of daily consumption of pomegranate juice.

At the beginning of the study a team of researchers tested the volunteers' blood pressure and asked them to describe their feelings towards their job.

After drinking 500ml of pomegranate juice everyday for two weeks the participants said they were more enthusiastic, inspired, proud and active at work.

They all also reported that they were less distressed, nervous, guilty and ashamed and full results of the study will be presented at an international conference in Barcelona in October.

Research Scientist, Dr Emad Al-Dujaili who led the study said: "On the basis of these findings there is a justified argument for busy workers to drink pomegranate juice to help alleviate chronic stress and maintain good health."

"There is a growing body of evidence that pomegranate juice delivers wide-ranging health benefits that merit further research."

"It is very rare indeed for an all-natural juice to offer the range of health benefits that we are seeing in pomegranate juice," Al-Dujaili added.

An earlier study by Queen Margaret University researchers found that pomegranate juice may redistribute weight around the body, moving fat away from stomachs and muffin tops.

The Benefits of Pomegranate Fruit Leaves For Health

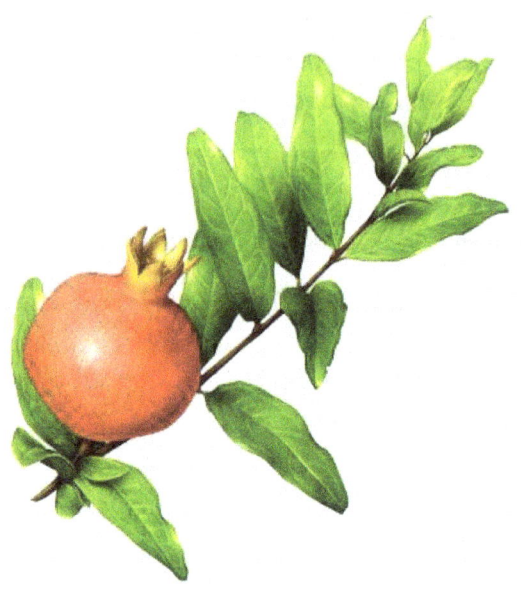

Pomegranate plants can actually be exploited everything, such as leaves, seeds, fruit peel and roots.

Health Benefits of Pomegranate For Leaves

1. Able to overcome insomnia

Pomegranate leaves may overcome insomnia (difficulty sleeping). How to make: take 3 grams of pomegranate leaf and washed, then boiled in two cups of water to the remaining half. After that, taken at the time of going to sleep.

2. Can cope with abdominal pain

Pomegranate leaf can also cope with abdominal pain. You can consume pomegranate leaf tea, can help digestion and can cope with abdominal pain.

3. Can cope with dysentery

Pomegranate leaves may also be overcome dysentery. It was thanks to the content in the leaves of pomegranate anti-bacterial, how to make: you can consume fruit juice and mixed with pomegranate leaf, can help to overcome dysentery and gastrointestinal infections.

4. It can relieve the symptoms of jaundice

Pomegranate leaves can also relieve symptoms of jaundice. You can use powdered leaves of the pomegranate. How to prepare: prepare 3 grams of powdered pomegranate leaves, then boiled with water.

5. Can treat a cough

Pomegranate leaf can also treat a cough. How to make: take leaves of pomegranate and dried, then boiled with water and mixed with black pepper and leaf buds.

6. Can be overcome thrush

Pomegranate leaves may also address canker sores. Thrush is a disturbance occurs in the lips, mouth or tongue. Marked with a wound in the area, which can cause pain or tenderness. How to cope: by means of rinsing with water decoction of the leaves of pomegranate.

7. Can cope with rectal prolapse

Pomegranate leaves may also address rectal prolapse. How to cope: soak with water decoction of the leaves of pomegranate, which has been mixed with alum and filtered.

Other Benefits of Pomegranate Fruit For Body Healing

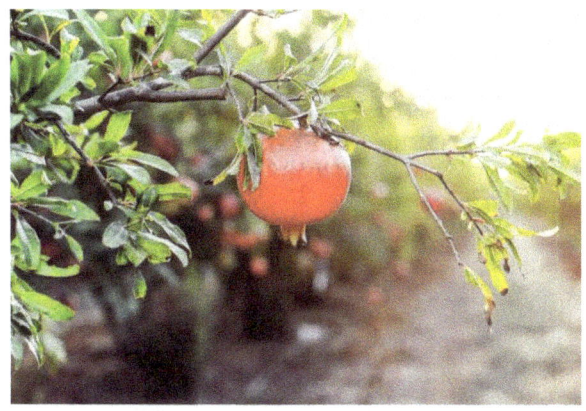

Here are some of the potential benefits of pomegranate.

1. Antioxidants

Pomegranates have been eaten throughout history for their health benefits. Nowadays, the juice of this fruit is a popular part of healthy diets.

Pomegranate seeds get their vibrant red hue from polyphenols. These chemicals are powerful antioxidants.

Pomegranate juice contains higher levels of antioxidants than most other fruit juices. It also has three times more antioxidants than red wine and green tea. The antioxidants in pomegranate juice can help remove free radicals, protect cells from damage, and reduce inflammation.

2. Vitamin C

The juice of a single pomegranate has more than 40 percent of your daily requirement of vitamin C. Vitamin C can be broken down when pasteurized, so opt for homemade or fresh pomegranate juice to get the most of the nutrient.

3. Cancer prevention

Pomegranate juice recently made a splash when researchers found that it may help stop the growth of prostate cancer cells. Despite multiple studies on the effects of the juice on prostate cancer, results are still preliminary.

While there haven't been long-term studies with humans that prove that pomegranate juice prevents cancer or reduces the risk, adding it to your diet certainly can't hurt. There have been encouraging results in studies so far, and bigger studies are now being done.

4. Alzheimer's disease protection

The antioxidants in the juice and their high concentration are believed to stall the progress of Alzheimer disease and protect memory.

5. Digestion

Pomegranate juice can reduce inflammation in the gut and improve digestion. It may be beneficial for people with Crohn's disease, ulcerative colitis, and other inflammatory bowel diseases.

While there are conflicting beliefs and research on whether pomegranate juice helps or worsens diarrhea, most doctors recommend avoiding it until you are feeling better and your symptoms have subsided.

6. Anti-inflammatory

Pomegranate juice is a powerful anti-inflammatory because of its high concentration of antioxidants. It can help reduce inflammation throughout the body and prevent oxidative stress and damage.

7. Arthritis

Flavonols in pomegranate juice may help block the inflammation that contributes to osteoarthritis and cartilage damage. The juice is currently being studiedTrusted Source for its potential effects on osteoporosis, rheumatoid arthritis, and other types of arthritis and joint inflammation.

8. Heart disease

Pomegranate juice is in the running as the most heart-healthy juice. It appears to protect the heart and arteries.

Small studies have shown that the juice improves blood flow and keeps the arteries from becoming stiff and thick. It may also slow the growth of plaque and buildup of cholesterol in the arteries. But pomegranate may react negatively with blood pressure and cholesterol medications like statins.

Be sure to talk with your doctor before indulging in the juice or taking a pomegranate extract supplement.

9. Blood pressure

Drinking pomegranate juice daily may also help lower systolic blood pressure. A comprehensive review of randomized controlled trials stated that it would be beneficial for heart health to include pomegranate juice daily.

10. Antiviral

Between the vitamin C and other immune-boosting nutrients like vitamin E, pomegranate juice can prevent illness and fight off infection. Pomegranates have also been shown to be antibacterial and antiviral in lab tests. They are being studied for their effects on common infections and viruses.

11. Vitamin-Rich

In addition to vitamin C and vitamin E, pomegranate juice is a good source of folate, potassium, and vitamin K.

Whether you decide to add pomegranate to your daily diet or just sip on it every now and then, check the label to ensure that it is 100 percent pure pomegranate juice, without added sugar. Or, juice it fresh.

12. Memory

Drinking 8 ounces of pomegranate juice a daily may improve learning and memory, according to a recent study.

13. Sexual performance and fertility

Pomegranate juice's concentration of antioxidants and ability to impact oxidative stress make it a potential fertility aid. Oxidative stress has been shown to cause sperm dysfunction and decrease fertility in women.

The juice has also been shown to help reduce oxidative stress in the placenta. But researchers don't yet know the exact benefits this may provide. Drinking pomegranate juice can also increase testosterone levels in men and women, one of the main hormones behind sex drive.

14. Endurance and sports performance

Move over, tart cherry and beet juice. Pomegranate juice may be the new sport performance enhancer. The juice may help reduce soreness and improve strength recovery. It also decreases oxidative damage caused by exercise.

15. Diabetes

Pomegranate was traditionally used as a remedy for diabetes in the Middle East and India. While much is still unknown about the effects of pomegranate on diabetes, it may help decrease insulin resistance and lower blood sugar.

Epilog

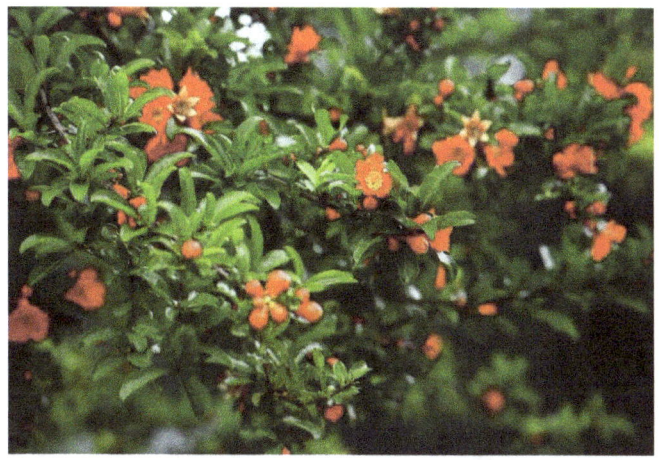

Green juice isn't the only healthy option out there.

Adding pomegranate fruit juice to your diet may reduce your risk for chronic disease and inflammation.

It's also a great way to get the fruit's nutrients and a boost of antioxidants.

References

"Pomegranate". Department of Plant Sciences, University of California at Davis, College of Agricultural & Environmental Sciences, Davis, CA. 2014

"Pomegranate Afghan Agriculture". University of California at Davis, International Programs. 2013

Seeram, N. P.; Schulman, R. N.; Heber, D., eds. (2006). Pomegranates: Ancient Roots to Modern Medicine. CRC Press.

Morton, J. F. (1987). "Pomegranate, Punica granatum L". Fruits of Warm Climates. Purdue New Crops Profile.

Holland, D.; Hatib, K.; Bar-Ya'akov, I. (2009). "Pomegranate: Botany, Horticulture, Breeding" Horticultural Reviews.

The Benefits of Pomegranate Fruit from Jannah Paradise For Mental Health & Body Healing

Jannah Firdaus Mediapro

The Benefits of Pomegranate Fruit from Jannah Paradise For Mental Health & Body Healing

www.ingramcontent.com/pod-product-compliance
Lightning Source LLC
LaVergne TN
LVHW020420070526
838199LV00055B/3676